Assessing Community Health Programs

A Participant's Manual and Workbook

Using LQAS for Baseline Surveys and Regular Monitoring

Joseph J. Valadez, PhD, MPH, ScD
William Weiss, MA
Corey Leburg, MHS
Robb Davis, PhD, MPH

Teaching-aids At Low Cost (TALC), St Albans (UK)

Published by:
Teaching-aids At Low Cost.
PO Box 49 St Albans Herts AL1 5TX UK

www.talcuk.org

ISBN: 0-9544894-2-X

All rights reserved.

First Published 2003
Text © Joseph J. Valadez
Illustrations © Hesperian Foundation

TALC (Teaching-aids At Low Cost) is a UK registered charity (no: 279858) and a Company limited by guarantee registered in England (no: 1477636) which supplies teaching-aids and books to raise standards of health care and reduce poverty worldwide.

Although every effort has been made to ensure the completeness and accuracy of the information contained in this publication, TALC cannot be held responsible for any recommendations contained therein or any errors that may have inadvertently occurred. TALC shall not, therefore, be liable under any circumstances whatsoever, for any damages suffered as a result of any such errors, omissions or recommendations arising from the use of this publication.

Cover design: Hesperian Foundation

Graphics and Design: Hesperian Foundation

Copy Editing: Freedom From Hunger

Structure, Training and Typesetting: Valadez, Weiss, Leburg, and Davis

Printed by: Photolit Printing Ltd. [St Albans. England]

We dedicate this book to community health workers and local program supervisors working to improve the health of people in communities throughout the world. We also dedicate this book to our mothers—special people in our lives.

Copyright © 2003 by Joseph J. Valadez. All rights reserved.
First Printing January 2003

NGOs, PVOs, International Organizations, Ministries of Health, universities may reproduce these materials for educational purposes or to improve health programs. None of these materials may be reproduced for commercial purposes without written permission.

This publication was made possible through support provided by the Bureau for Global Health, U.S. Agency for International Development, under the terms of Award No. HRN-A-00-98-00011-00. The opinions expressed herein are those of the authors and do not necessarily reflect the views of the U.S. Agency for International Development.

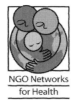 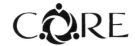

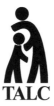

Teaching-aids At Low Cost (TALC)
PO Box 49
St Albans, Herts
AL1 5TX UK
Tel: 00 44 (0) 1727 853869
Fax: 00 44 (0) 1727 846852
Email: info@talcuk.org
Website: www.talcuk.org

TABLE OF CONTENTS

A Participant's Manual and Workbook: Using LQAS for Baseline Surveys and Regular Monitoring

MODULE ONE: Why should I do a survey and why should I use the LQAS method?   Page PM-5

Session 1: Introducing Participants and the Training/Survey   page PM-6

> Overhead #1—Getting to Know Each Other
> Overhead #2—Purpose of the LQAS Workshop
> Overhead #3—Skills to be Learned
> Overhead #4—Overview of the LQAS Training
> Overhead #5—Abbreviated Training Schedule/Agenda
> Overhead #6—Defining Catchment Area and Supervision Areas

Session 2: Uses of Surveys   page PM-14

> Overhead #7—What is Coverage?
> Overhead #8—What Surveys Can Show You
> Overhead #9—NGO Program Area: Scenario 1
> Overhead #10—NGO Program Area: Scenario 2
> Overhead #11—NGO Program Area: Scenario 3
> Overhead #12—Using Survey Data
> Overhead #13—Uses of Surveys

Session 3: Random Sampling   page PM-21

> Overhead #14—Why Random Sample?

Session 4: Using LQAS Sampling for Surveys   page PM-22

> Overhead #15—NGO Program Area: Scenario 4
> Overhead #16—LQAS Sampling Results
> Overhead #17—The LQAS Table
> Overhead #18—What a Sample of 19 Can Tell Us
> Overhead #19—What a Sample of 19 Cannot Tell Us
> Overhead #20—Why Use a Sample of 19?

Session 5: Using LQAS for Baseline Surveys   page PM-28

> Overhead #21—Five Supervision Areas and One Indicator
> Overhead #22—LQAS Concepts for Baseline Surveys
> Overhead #23—Five Supervision Areas and One Indicator: Participant Worksheet
> Overhead #24—Supervision Area A and Five Indicators
> Overhead #25—Comparing Supervision Areas A, B, C, D, and E

MODULE TWO: Where should I conduct my survey?   Page PM-33

Session 1: Identifying Interview Locations   page PM-34

> Overhead #1—Identifying Locations for Interviews
> Overhead #2—List of Communities and Total Population for a Supervision Area
> Overhead #3—Calculate the Cumulative Population
> Overhead #4—Calculate the Sampling Interval
> Overhead #5—Random Number Table
> Overhead #6—Identify the Location of Each of the 19 Interviews in a Supervision Area: Work Sheet
> Overhead #7—LQAS Sampling Frame for a Supervision Area

MODULE THREE: Whom should I interview?   Page PM-41

Session 1: Selecting Households   page PM-42

> Overhead #1—How to Assign Numbers to Households
> Overhead #2—Situation 2: Household List Not Available: Size About 30
> Overhead #3—Situation 3: Household List Not Available: Size Greater Than 30
> Overhead #4—Group of 27 Households Numbered for Random Selection of 1 Household

Session 2: Selecting Respondents   page PM-46

> Overhead #5— Rules for Identifying Respondents
> Overhead #6— Household Composition Scenarios

Session 3: Field Practical for Numbering and Selecting Households   page PM-51

> Overhead #7—Process for Field Practical

MODULE FOUR: What questions do I ask and how should I ask them? — Page PM-52

Session 1: Reviewing the Survey Questionnaires — page PM----
> No overheads

Session 2: Interviewing Skills — page PM-53
> Overhead #1—Why Interviewing is Important
> Overhead #2—Interview Etiquette
> Overhead #3—Effective Interviewing Techniques

Session 3: Field Practical for Interviewing — page PM---
> No overheads

Session 4: Planning for the Data Collection/Survey — page PM-56
> HANDOUT - Survey Checklists

MODULE FIVE: What do I do with the information I have collected during the baseline survey? — Page PM-59

Session 1: Fieldwork Debriefing — page PM-60
> Overhead #1—Status Report on Data Collection from the NGO

Session 2: Tabulating Results — page PM-61
> Overhead #2—Result Tabulation Table
> HANDOUT— Tabulation Quality Checklist

Session 3: Analyzing Results — page PM-65
> Overhead #3—Summary Tabulation Sheet for Baseline Surveys
> Overhead #4—The LQAS Table
> Overhead #5—Defining Program Goals and Annual Targets
> Overhead #6—Monitoring Targets and Average Coverage Over Time: In a Catchment Area
> Overhead #7—How To Analyze Data and Identify Priorities Using the Summary Tables
> Overhead #8—Baseline Survey Report Format
> Overhead #9—Methodology
> Overhead #10—Main Findings
> Overhead #11—Action Plans/Goals/Coverage Targets for Key Indicators

MODULE SIX: What do I do with the information I have collected during regular monitoring? Page PM-74

Session 1: Fieldwork Debriefing page PM-75

> Overhead #1—Status Report on Data Collection from the NGO

Session 2: Tabulating Results page PM-76

> Overhead #2—Result Tabulation Table
> HANDOUT—Tabulation Quality Checklist

Session 3: Analyzing Results page PM-80

> Overhead #3—Summary Tabulation Sheet for Regular Monitoring
> Overhead #4—The LQAS Table
> Overhead #5—Defining Program Goals and Annual Targets
> Overhead #6—How to Identify Priority SAs Using the Summary Tables During Regular Monitoring
> Overhead #7—Using LQAS to Assess One Indicator Over the Life of a Project
> Overhead #8—Monitoring Targets and Average Coverage Over Time: In a Catchment Area
> Overhead #9—How To Analyze Data and Identify Priorities Using the Summary Tables
> Overhead #10—Monitoring Survey Report Format
> Overhead #11—Methodology
> Overhead #12—Main Findings
> Overhead #13—Action Plans/Goals/Coverage Targets for Key Indicators

LQAS Table: Bring This Table With You to Use in the Field or for Easy Reference Page PM-91

MODULE ONE

Why should I do a survey and why should I use the LQAS method?

Session 1: Introducing Participants and the Training/Survey

Session 2: Uses of Surveys

Session 3: Random Sampling

Session 4: Using LQAS Sampling for Surveys

Session 5: Using LQAS for Baseline Surveys

Module One
Session 1
Overhead 1

Getting to Know Each Other

1. What organization are you from?

2. What is your position/what do you do?

3. What is your interest in doing surveys?

4. What kind of experience do you have with surveys?

Module One
Session 1
Overhead 2

Purpose of the LQAS Workshop

➤ Train participants in how to conduct surveys to collect data for establishing baselines and for regular monitoring.

➤ Train participants in how to analyze data to identify priorities for improving program coverage.

Module One
Session 1
Overhead 3

Skills to Be Learned

➢ **LQAS Sampling Methods**

➢ **Interviewing Techniques**

➢ **Data Tabulation and Analysis for Program Improvement**

Module One
Session 1
Overhead 4

Overview of the LQAS Training

PRE-SURVEY

Module 1. Why should I do a survey & why should I use the LQAS method?

1. Introducing participants and the training survey
2. Uses of surveys
3. Random Sampling
4. Using LQAS sampling for surveys
5. Using LQAS for baseline surveys

Module 2. Where should I conduct my survey?

1. Introducing interview locations

Module 3. Who should I interview?

1. Selecting households
2. Selecting respondents
3. Field practical for numbering and selecting households

CARRY OUT SURVEY

Module 4. What questions do I ask and how do I ask them?

1. Reviewing the survey questionnaires
2. Interviewing skills
3. Field practical for interviewing
4. Planning for the data collection/survey

POST-SURVEY

Module 5 or 6. What do I do with the information I have collected?

1. Field work debriefing
2. Tabulating results
3. Analyzing results

Participant's Manual, Module 1

PM-9

Module One
Session 1
Overhead 5

Abbreviated Agenda for Modules 1-4: Sampling and Data Collection Workshop

Day 1
Morning
- Opening and Introductions
- Uses of Surveys
- Random Sampling
- Using LQAS

Afternoon
- Using LQAS continued
- Identifying Interview Locations – communities
- Selecting Households

Day 2
Morning
- Selecting Respondents
- Field Practical for Numbering and Selecting Households

Afternoon
- Review and Discuss Field Practical
- Review Survey Questionnaires

Day 3
Morning
- Review Survey Questionnaires cont.
- Interviewing Techniques

Afternoon
- Field Practical for Interviewing

Day 4
Morning
- Review and Discuss Field Practical
- Improving Interviewing Skills
- Develop Final Plans for Data Collection

Afternoon
- Develop Final Plans for Data Collection cont.
- Workshop Certificates Awarded and Closing

Module One
Session 1
Overhead 5 cont.

Abbreviated Agenda for Module 5 (Baselines): Tabulation and Data Analysis Workshop

Day 1
Morning
    Opening and Welcome Back
    Field Work Debriefing
    Lessons learned During the Data Collection
    Agreement on Correct Answers on Questionnaires
    How to Use the Tabulation Tables

Afternoon
    Calculating Average Coverage and its Importance
    Two Exercises: Using the Tabulation Tables
    Begin Tabulation in Stages

Day 2
Morning
    Continue Tabulation in Stages

Afternoon
    Continue Tabulation in Stages

Day 3
Morning
    Continue Tabulation in Stages

Afternoon
    Continue Tabulation in Stages
    How to Analyze LQAS Data and Identify Priorities
    Preparing a Baseline Report
    Next Steps and the Future

Module One
Session 1
Alternative Overhead 5 cont.

Abbreviated Agenda for Module 6 (Monitoring and Evaluation): Tabulation and Data Analysis Workshop

Day 1
Morning
- Opening and Welcome Back
- Field Work Debriefing
- Lessons Learned During the Data Collection
- Agreement on Correct Answers on Questionnaires
- How to Use the Tabulation Tables

Afternoon
- Calculating Average Coverage and its Importance
- Reviewing Performance Benchmarks for the Project
- Two Exercises: Using the Tabulation Tables
- Begin Tabulation in Stages

Day 2
Morning
- Continue Tabulation in Stages

Afternoon
- Continue Tabulation in Stages

Day 3
Morning
- Continue Tabulation in Stages

Afternoon
- Continue Tabulation in Stages
- How to Analyze LQAS Data and Identify Priorities Using Average Coverage and Performance Benchmarks
- Preparing a Monitoring and/or Evaluation Report
- Next Steps and the Future

Module One
Session 1
Overhead 6

Defining Catchment Area and Supervision Areas

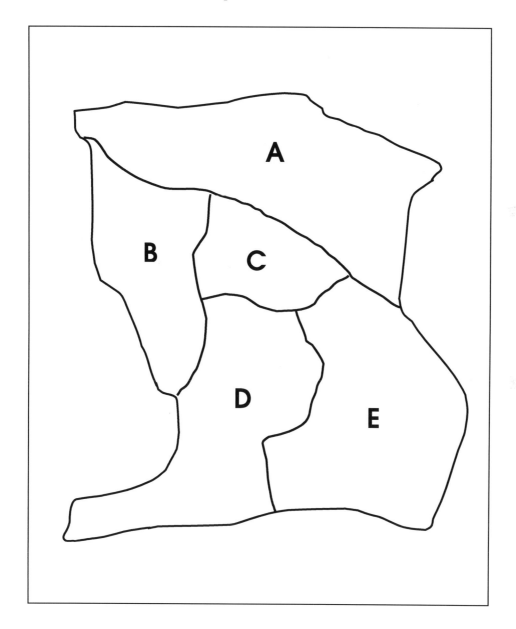

Together, A, B, C, D, and E represent the <u>Catchment Area</u>,

A, B, C, D, and E represent 5 <u>Supervision Areas</u>.

Module One
Session 2
Overhead 7

What is Coverage?

An important use of surveys is to measure coverage.

➤ **What is coverage?**

➤ **Why is it important to know about coverage?**

Module One
Session 2
Overhead 8

What Surveys Can Show You

Surveys can help you identify the level of coverage of the program area as a whole, AND if there are:

> ➤ *<u>large</u>* differences in coverage regarding health knowledge and practices among supervision areas

> ➤ *<u>little</u>* difference in coverage regarding health knowledge and practices among supervision areas

Module One
Session 2
Overhead 9

NGO PROGRAM: Scenario One (1)
Supervision Areas: A - E
Indicator: Percent of women (15-49) who know 2 or more ways to prevent HIV transmission.

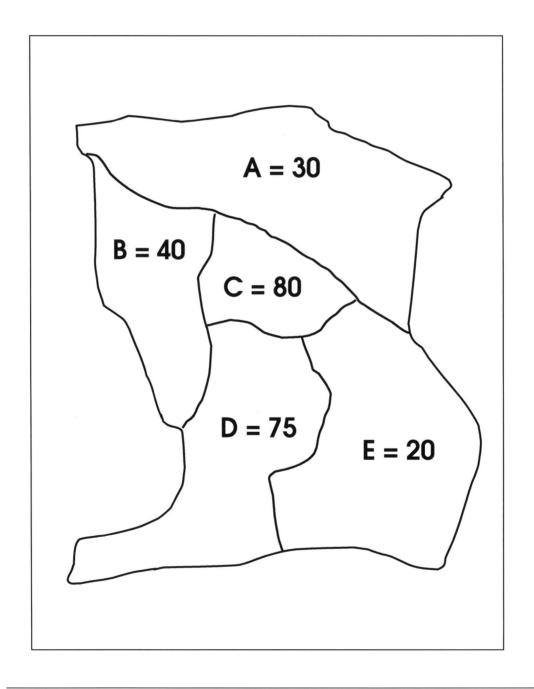

Module One
Session 2
Overhead 10

NGO PROGRAM: Scenario Two (2)
Supervision Areas: A - E
Indicator: Percent of women (15-49) who know 2 or more ways to prevent HIV transmission.

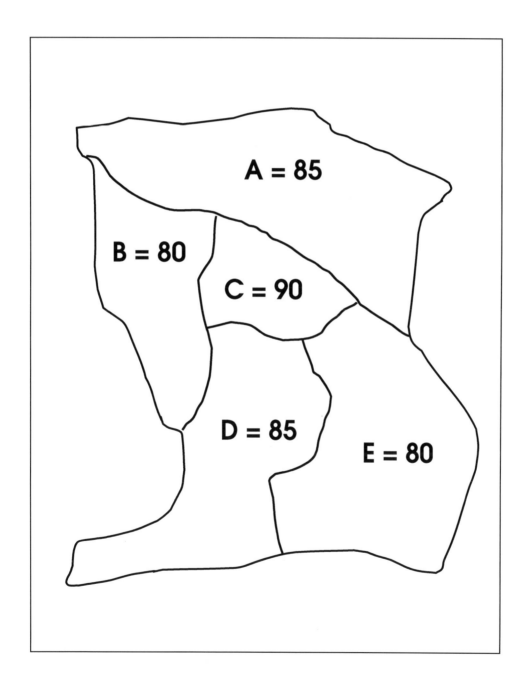

Participant's Manual, Module 1   **PM-17**

Module One
Session 2
Overhead 11

NGO PROGRAM: Scenario Three (3)
Supervision Areas: A - E
Indicator: Percent of women (15-49) who know 2 or more ways to prevent HIV transmission.

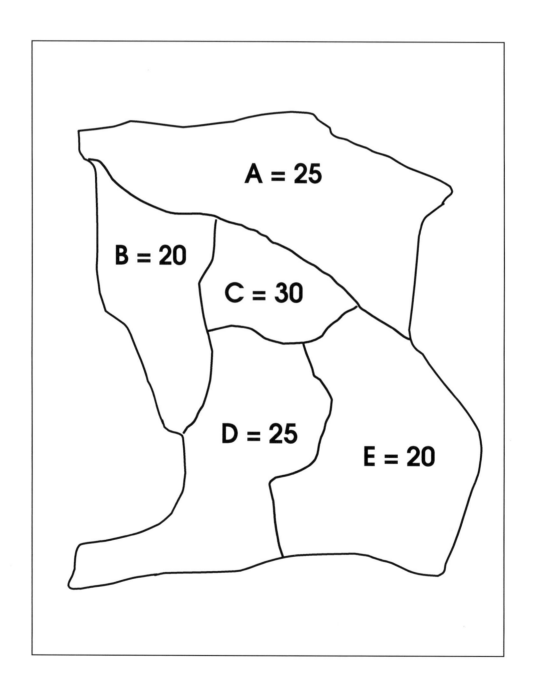

Module One
Session 2
Overhead 12

Using Survey Data

Indicator: Percent of women (15-49) who know at least two ways to prevent HIV transmission

Supervision Area	Possible Scenarios		
	Scenario One (1) True Coverage (%)	Scenario Two (2) True Coverage (%)	Scenario Three (3) True Coverage (%)
A	30	85	25
B	40	80	20
C	80	90	30
D	75	85	25
E	20	80	20

Analysis:

Look only at the true coverage figures within your assigned scenario (1, 2 or 3):

1. Discuss for a few minutes the differences in coverage among the 5 supervision areas *within your scenario*:
   - What is the difference in coverage among the 5 supervision areas?
   - How different is this? Very different? Little difference?

2. Does coverage for the overall program area appear HIGH, LOW, or MIXED?

3. What may be possible reasons for why, in your scenario, the program area has this coverage?

4. What might you propose to do about HIV/AIDS in the program area?

Module One
Session 2
Overhead 13

Uses of Surveys

Identify health knowledge and practices with:

1. *Large* differences in coverage among supervision areas (SAs).

→ Identify the low-coverage SAs to be able to:
- learn causes of low coverage.

- focus our efforts and resources on these SAs.

- improve coverage of the whole NGO program area by improving coverage in these SAs.

→ Identify high-coverage SAs to be able to:
- study and learn what is working well.

- identify things that can be applied to other SAs.

2. *Little* difference in coverage among SAs.

→ If coverage is generally high, shift resources to improve other health knowledge and practices.

→ If coverage is generally low:
- learn causes of low coverage.

- identify/study other NGO program areas to learn what is working well.

- identify things that can be applied in your own program area.

Module One
Session 3
Overhead 14

Why Random Sample?

Sampling allows you to use the "*few*" to describe the "*whole*," and this:

> **Saves time**

and

> **Saves money**

Module One
Session 4
Overhead 15

NGO PROGRAM: Scenario Four (4)
Supervision Areas: A - E
Indicator: Percent of women (15-49) who know at least 2 ways to prevent HIV transmission.

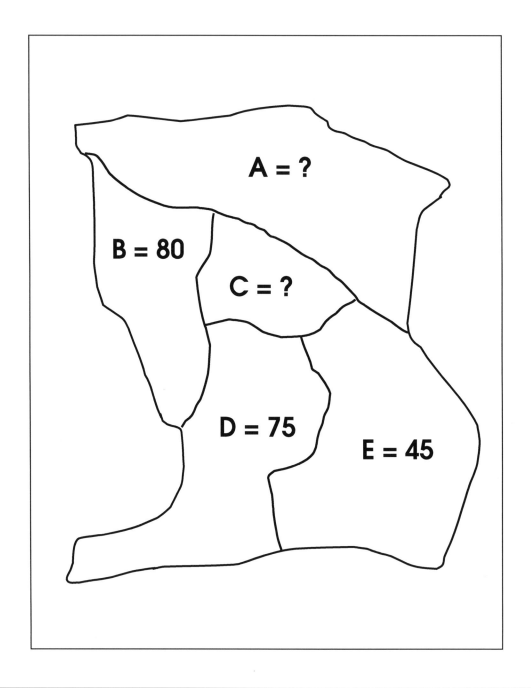

Module One
Session 4
Overhead 16

LQAS Sampling Results

Indicator: Percent of women (15-49) who know at least 2 ways to prevent HIV transmission.

	Supervision Areas: NGO Program Area	
	A	C
Sample	# Correct (green marbles)	# Correct (green marbles)
1		
2		
3		
4		
5		

Verify "coverage" in the bag for <u>SA A</u> → $\dfrac{\text{Total green marbles in the bag}}{\text{Total green and red marbles in the bag}}$ = ☐/☐ = _____%

Verify "coverage" in the bag for <u>SA C</u> → $\dfrac{\text{Total green marbles in the bag}}{\text{Total green and red marbles in the bag}}$ = ☐/☐ = _____%

Module One
Session 4
Overhead 17

LQAS Table: Decision Rules for Sample Sizes of 12-30 and Coverage Targets/Average of 10%-95%

Sample Size*	Average Coverage (Baselines) / Annual Coverage Target (Monitoring and Evaluation)																	
	10%	15%	20%	25%	30%	35%	40%	45%	50%	55%	60%	65%	70%	75%	80%	85%	90%	95%
12	N/A	N/A	1	1	2	2	3	4	5	5	6	7	7	8	8	9	10	11
13	N/A	N/A	1	1	2	3	3	4	5	6	6	7	8	8	9	10	11	11
14	N/A	N/A	1	1	2	3	4	4	5	6	7	8	8	9	10	11	11	12
15	N/A	N/A	1	2	2	3	4	5	6	6	7	8	9	10	10	11	12	13
16	N/A	N/A	1	2	2	3	4	5	6	7	8	9	9	10	11	12	13	14
17	N/A	N/A	1	2	2	3	4	5	6	7	8	9	10	11	12	13	14	15
18	N/A	N/A	1	2	2	3	5	6	7	8	9	10	11	11	12	13	14	16
19	N/A	N/A	1	2	3	4	5	6	7	8	9	10	11	12	13	14	15	16
20	N/A	N/A	1	2	3	4	5	6	7	8	9	11	12	13	14	15	16	17
21	N/A	N/A	1	2	3	4	5	6	8	9	10	11	12	13	14	16	17	18
22	N/A	N/A	1	2	3	4	5	7	8	9	10	12	13	14	15	16	18	19
23	N/A	N/A	1	2	3	4	6	7	8	10	11	12	13	14	16	17	18	20
24	N/A	N/A	1	2	3	4	6	7	9	10	11	13	14	15	16	18	19	21
25	N/A	1	2	2	4	5	6	8	9	10	12	13	14	16	17	18	20	21
26	N/A	1	2	3	4	5	6	8	9	11	12	14	15	16	18	19	21	22
27	N/A	1	2	3	4	5	7	8	10	11	13	14	15	17	18	20	21	23
28	N/A	1	2	3	4	5	7	8	10	12	13	15	16	18	19	21	22	24
29	N/A	1	2	3	4	5	7	9	10	12	13	15	17	18	20	21	23	25
30	N/A	1	2	3	4	5	7	9	11	12	14	16	17	19	20	22	24	26

N/A: *not applicable*, meaning LQAS can not be used in this assessment because the coverage is either too low or too high to assess an SA. This table assumes the lower threshold is 30 percentage points below the upper threshold.

▨ : shaded cells indicate where *alpha or beta* errors are ≥ 10%.

▧ : hashed cells indicate where *alpha or beta* errors are > 15%.

Module One
Session 4
Overhead 18

What a Random Sample of 19 Can Tell Us

➤ Good for deciding what are the higher-performing supervision areas to learn from

➤ Good for deciding what are the lower-performing supervision areas

➤ Good for differentiating knowledge/practices that have high coverage from those of low coverage

➤ Good for setting priorities among supervision areas with large differences in coverage

➤ Good for setting priorities among knowledge/practices within an SA

(if one intervention is high but the other is low, we would concentrate on the low-coverage intervention)

Module One
Session 4
Overhead 19

What a Random Sample of 19 Cannot Tell Us

➤ **Not good for calculating exact coverage in an SA (but can be used to calculate coverage for an entire program)**

➤ **Not good for setting priorities among supervision areas that have little difference in coverage among them**

Module One
Session 4
Overhead 20

Why Use a Random Sample of 19?

- **A sample of 19 provides an acceptable level of error for making management decisions; at least 92% of the time it correctly identifies SAs that have reached their coverage target.**

- **Samples larger than 19 have practically the same statistical precision as 19. They do not result in better information, and they cost more.**

Module One
Session 5
Overhead 21

Five Supervision Areas & One Indicator

SUPERVISION AREA: A, B, C, D or E			
Indicator: Women who know at least 2 ways to prevent HIV transmission	**# Correct**	**Coverage Estimate = 65.3%**	**Equal to or Above Average? Yes or No**
Supervision Area A	12		Yes
Supervision Area B	9		No
Supervision Area C	16	**Decision Rule = 11**	Yes
Supervision Area D	11		Yes
Supervision Area E	14		Yes

1. Add Number Correct in all SAs: 12 + 9 + 16 + 11 +14 = **62**
   Add all Samples Sizes: 19 + 19 + 19+ 19 + 19 = **95**
   Coverage Estimate = Average Coverage = 62/95 = **65.3%** = **70%**
   (Round upward to the nearest interval of 5 to find the Decision Rule)

2. Use table to find Decision Rule.

3. Is coverage in Supervision Areas generally equal to or below average? Yes or No?

4. Can you identify Supervision Areas that are your priorities?

5. If yes, which are they? If not, why can't you identify them?

LQAS Concepts for Baseline Surveys

➢ "Average Coverage" for a question/indicator is the number of people in the sample who responded correctly to a question divided by the total number of people responding to that question.

➢ The "Decision Rule" tells you whether an individual supervision area reaches the average coverage or is below average coverage.

Module One
Session 5
Overhead 23

Five Supervision Areas & One Indicator: Participant Worksheet – For Baseline Surveys

Indicator: Women who used condoms each time with intercourse	# Correct	Coverage Estimate =	Equal to or Above Average? Yes or No
Supervision Area A	7		
Supervision Area B	3		
Supervision Area C	2	Decision Rule (Using the LQAS Table) =	
Supervision Area D	13		
Supervision Area E	14		

Questions:

1. For baseline surveys, add number correct in all SAs:

    7 + 3 + 2 + 13 + 14 = 39

    Add all sample sizes: 19 + 19 + 19 + 19 + 19 = _____

    Average coverage = _____ / _____ = _____ %

2. What is the Decision Rule?

3. Is coverage is SAs generally equal to or above average? Yes or No?

4. Can you identify Supervision Areas that are your priorities?

5. If yes, which are they? If not, why can't you identify them?

PM-30 Participant's Manual, Module 1

Module One
Session 5
Overhead 24

Supervision Area A & Five Indicators

	Indicators	# Correct	Coverage Estimate	Decision Rule	Equal to or Above Average? Yes or No
1	Women who used condoms each time with intercourse	7	45%	6	
2	Men who used condoms each time with intercourse	4	20%		
3	Women who know how HIV is transmitted	4	45%		
4	Men who know how HIV is transmitted	13	65%		
5	Women who know where to get tested for HIV	6	30%		

Questions:

1. Can you identify indicators that are your priorities?

2. If yes, which indicators are they? If not, why can't you identify them?

Module One
Session 5
Overhead 25

Comparing Supervision Areas A, B, C, D, & E
(for baseline survey)

	Indicators	Supervision Area				
		A	B	C	D	E
1	Women who used condoms each time with intercourse				Y	Y
2	Men who used condoms each time with intercourse	Y	Y	Y	N	Y
3	Women who know how HIV is transmitted	N	N	Y	N	Y
4	Men who know how HIV is transmitted	Y	Y	N	N	Y
5	Women who know where to get tested for HIV	Y	Y	Y	N	Y

Questions:

1. Which Supervision Area(s) appears to be performing the best for all 5 indicators: A, B, C, D, or E? ____

2. Which SA(s) appears to need the most support for their overall program: A, B, C, D, or E? ____

3. Which indicator(s) needs improvement across most of the catchment area? ____

4. Which indicator(s) needs improvement in only a few SAs? ____

5. For these weaker indicators :
   - Which SA(s) needs special attention? ____

   - Which SA(s) would you visit to learn possible ways to improve these weaker indicator? ____

PM-32   Participant's Manual, Module 1

MODULE TWO

Where should I conduct my survey?

Session 1: Identifying Interview Locations

Module Two
Session 1
Overhead 1

Identifying Locations for Interviews

Step 1. List communities and total population.

Step 2. Calculate the cumulative population.

Step 3. Calculate the sampling interval.

Step 4. Choose a random number.

Step 5. Beginning with the random number, use the sampling interval to identify communities for the 19 sets of interviews.

List of Communities and Total Population for a Supervision Area

Name of Community	Total Population
Pagai	548
Santai	730
Serina	686
Mulrose	280
Fanta	1256
Bagia	684
Rostam	919
Mt. Sil	1374
Livton	1136
Farry	544
Tunis	193
Pulau	375
Sasarota	333
Pingra	3504
Kanata	336
Sirvish	2115
Balding	258
Rescuut	678
Krista	207
Manalopa	1162
Garafa	408
Spiltar	455
Masraf	978
Abrama	335
Junagadh	541
Singri	725
Kalarata	355
Ichimota	498
Chaplar	347
Sr. Kitt	186
Nevis	1346
TOTAL	**23489**

Module Two
Session 1
Overhead 3

Calculate the Cumulative Population

of Community	Total Population	Cumulative Population
Pagai	548	548
Santai	730	
Serina	686	
Mulrose	280	
Fanta	1256	3500
Bagia	684	4184
Rostam	919	5103
Mt. Sil	1374	6477
Livton	1136	7610
Farry	544	8154
Tunis	193	8347
Pulau	375	8722
Sasarota	333	9055
Pingra	3504	12559
Kanata	336	12895
Sirvish	2115	15010
Balding	258	15268
Rescuut	678	15946
Krista	207	16153
Manalopa	1162	17315
Garafa	408	17723
Spiltar	455	18178
Masraf	978	
Abrama	335	
Junagadh	541	
Singri	725	
Kalarata	355	
Ichimota	498	
Chaplar	347	
Sr. Kitt	186	
Nevis	1346	
TOTAL	**23489**	

Module Two
Session 1
Overhead 4

Calculate the Sampling Interval

Name of Community	Total Population	Cumulative Population
Pagai	548	548
Santai	730	1278
Serina	686	1964
Mulrose	280	2244
Fanta	1256	3500
Bagia	684	4184
Rostam	919	5103
Mt. Sil	1374	6477
Livton	1136	7610
Farry	544	8154
Tunis	193	8347
Pulau	375	8722
Sasarota	333	9055
Pingra	3504	12559
Kanata	336	12895
Sirvish	2115	15010
Balding	258	15268
Rescuut	678	15946
Krista	207	16153
Manalopa	1162	17315
Garafa	408	17723
Spiltar	455	18178
Masraf	978	19156
Abrama	335	19491
Junagadh	541	20032
Singri	725	20757
Kalarata	355	21112
Ichimota	498	21610
Chaplar	347	21957
Sr. Kitt	186	22143
Nevis	1346	23489
TOTAL	23489	--

Sampling Interval = Total Cumulative Population/19 = ?

Module Two
Session 1
Overhead 5

A Random Number Table

```
87172 43062 39719 10020 32722 86545 86985 04962 54546 23138 62135 55870 97083 67875
28900 50851 30543 89185 16747 95104 49852 26467 58869 79053 06894 23975 34902 23587
86248 71156 55044 13045 33161 95604 57876 23367 10768 78193 60477 70307 06498 48793
10531 51391 41884 69759 32741 70072 01902 96656 90584 59263 49995 27235 40055 20917
02481 90230 81978 39127 93335 74259 25856 52838 49847 69042 85964 78159 40374 49658
23988 13019 78830 17069 58267 69796 94329 34050 25622 55349 10403 93790 77631 74261
37137 47689 82466 24243 10756 54009 44053 74870 28352 66389 38729 80349 50509 56465
38230 82039 34158 90149 82948 60686 27962 39306 53826 47852 76144 38812 76939 03119
98745 08288 19108 84791 58470 59415 45456 44839 86274 25091 42809 56707 47169 95273
44653 58412 91751 14954 87949 81399 51105 29718 82780 11262 23712 99782 42829 26308
88386 66621 16648 19217 52375 05417 26136 05952 71958 25744 52021 20225 01377 47012
50660 58138 01695 69351 25445 20797 74079 60851 47634 36633 93999 96345 58484 12506
36732 74234 84240 46924 62744 39238 78397 60869 26426 55588 56963 59506 17293 45096
34187 78277 83678 34754 46616 45250 25291 04999 19717 60324 66915 03473 98329 82447
26095 98131 79362 39530 53870 87445 26277 90551 28604 39865 40686 05435 74511 69866
00067 74289 20706 74076 28206 36960 09231 82988 57062 35331 08212 68111 52199 05065
42104 26434 30953 15259 76676 63339 75664 23993 63538 34968 47655 44553 61982 13296
82580 46580 87292 23226 21865 60338 04115 33807 38395 98484 40387 69877 24910 13317
89266 14764 17681 68663 66030 12931 17372 35601 63805 55739 42705 30549 31697 33478
47100 92329 89435 69974 40783 52649 93444 41317 02749 19052 34647 92814 88046 34020
59566 26527 44706 85670 96223 36275 82013 82673 60955 62617 90214 24589 59715 57612
10946 24676 66513 56743 96911 89042 08263 70753 89045 39189 04306 06090 94515 17772
34013 69250 27977 84597 55192 65088 55739 35953 18533 39339 78037 32827 68269 69218
21606 11751 30073 71431 53569 27865 90215 34772 21779 11734 64313 49764 30816 56852
56620 92612 77157 90231 90144 29781 01683 52503 60080 73703 70080 80686 47379 33279
49238 90475 84356 87159 21222 40106 02671 52684 38514 68434 16407 58164 13341 48142
50738 21999 73539 51802 78179 27872 57937 29696 67783 29373 96563 74619 77099 17190
58761 21571 71692 19723 25088 10483 71430 47068 78378 80237 32113 09381 62931 29243
55335 71937 22025 33538 04648 74232 57839 62431 61835 04784 06732 34202 93497 72070
26515 31143 83795 78445 32869 31489 81587 90354 97672 70106 35008 37899 36246 97805
32625 36806 00082 26902 26250 28919 38054 49027 22209 42696 46980 17065 61288 30208
20311 96089 20141 30362 04980 32703 04202 91080 28660 89691 84660 73433 70169 11273
10941 73003 87930 85620 06956 38719 88711 61454 64076 13316 02203 54437 54306 78229
56982 46636 34070 30803 39095 80387 08971 25067 07377 70704 13629 68474 99229 05535
14661 10670 15811 00454 81124 46977 89983 48836 48182 17054 06344 24267 16686 21401
52760 78118 23277 29760 00099 97325 54762 43117 73199 19621 24599 11030 64809 35088
48874 20831 02286 73635 93771 54264 49801 22653 01524 84621 91023 64028 29278 15987
44817 77408 48447 25934 22912 43086 68126 92970 91833 26418 72454 97636 94593 07880
17896 79375 70883 70135 21589 51181 71969 32951 35036 17219 27357 96517 55307 84470
27166 22347 92146 92189 16301 15747 72837 59174 75024 39459 54910 95335 95013 47068
13665 30490 63583 73098 19976 03001 94645 40476 43617 85698 66512 42759 20973 98759
58644 73840 08103 97926 57340 63077 08114 10031 35668 21740 33787 44756 20527 65367
72570 36278 06602 56406 85679 85529 08576 50874 59706 01019 29980 56742 05356 04810
92041 68829 02163 59918 83041 71241 90678 79835 86324 13075 29913 99831 25688 53648
71240 74119 53090 23693 14007 90107 68804 54927 68964 26535 28184 21630 12362 67990
```

Module Two
Session 1
Overhead 6

Identify the Location of Each of the 19 Interviews in a Supervision Area: Worksheet

Random Number = 622   Sampling Interval = 1236.26

LQAS No.	Calculation	Interview Location
1.	Random Number = Location Number 1	**622**
2.	RN + Sampling Interval = Location Number 2	622+1236.26= **1858.26**
3.	Interview Location Number 2 + Sampling Interval	1858.26+1236.26= **3094.52**
4.	Interview Location Number 3 + Sampling Interval	3094.52+1236.26= **4330.78**
5.	Interview Location Number 4 + Sampling Interval	
6.	Interview Location Number 5 + Sampling Interval	
7.	Interview Location Number 6 + Sampling Interval	
8.	Interview Location Number 7 + Sampling Interval	
9.	Interview Location Number 8 + Sampling Interval	
10.	Interview Location Number 9 + Sampling Interval	
11.	Interview Location Number 10 + Sampling Interval	
12.	Interview Location Number 11 + Sampling Interval	
13.	Interview Location Number 12 + Sampling Interval	
14.	Interview Location Number 13 + Sampling Interval	
15.	Interview Location Number 14 + Sampling Interval	
16.	Interview Location Number 15 + Sampling Interval	
17.	Interview Location Number 16 + Sampling Interval	
18.	Interview Location Number 17 + Sampling Interval	
19.	Interview Location Number 18 + Sampling Interval	

Module Two
Session 1
Overhead 7

LQAS Sampling Frame for a Supervision Area

Name of Community	Total Population	Cumulative Population	Interview Location Number	Number of Interviews
Pagai	548	548		
Santai	730	1278	622.00	
Serina	686	1964	1858.26	
Mulrose	280	2244		
Fanta	1256	3500	3094.52	
Bagia	684	4184		
Rostam	919	5103	4330.78	
Mt. Sil	1374	6477		
Livton	1136	7610		
Farry	544	8154		
Tunis	193	8347		
Pulau	375	8722		
Sasarota	333	9055		
Pingra	3504	12559		
Kanata	336	12895		
Sirvish	2115	15010	12984.6, 14220.86	
Balding	258	15268		
Rescuut	678	15946	15457.12	
Krista	207	16153		
Manalopa	1162	17315	16693.38	
Garafa	408	17723		
Spiltar	455	18178	17929.64	
Masraf	978	19156		
Abrama	335	19491	19165.90	
Junagadh	541	20032		
Singri	725	20757	20402.16	
Kalarata	355	21112		
Ichimota	498	21610		
Chaplar	347	21957	21638.42	
Sr. Kitt	186	22143		
Nevis	1346	23489	22874.68	
TOTAL	23489			19

MODULE THREE

Whom should I interview?

Session 1: Selecting Households

Session 2: Selecting Respondents

Session 3: Field Practical for Numbering and Selecting Households

Module Three
Session 1
Overhead 1

How to Assign Numbers to Households

IF:	THEN:
A complete household list is available (tax list, census, map)	Assign a number to each house… …Work is done!
If the community size is "about" 30 households or less	Make a household list or map with the location of each household (use assistance of a key informant from the community)… And then assign a number to each house… (… **Alternatively, you can use the "spin-the-bottle technique …"**) … Work is done!
If the community size is more than "about" 30 households	Subdivide the community into 2-5 sections with about the same number of households in each section. …Select one section at random… …If the section has more houses than you can easily count, subdivide into 2-5 sections again and select one at random. Continue doing this until few houses remain. …Make a house list or map with the location of each household (use an assistant or key informant from your community). Then assign a number to each house. (… **Alternatively, you can use the "spin the bottle technique …"**) …Work is done!

<u>Household</u> = group of persons who share the same kitchen or hearth; or, a group of persons who eat from the same cooking pot.

Module Three
Session 1
Overhead 2

Situation 2: Household List Not Available – Size 'About' 30

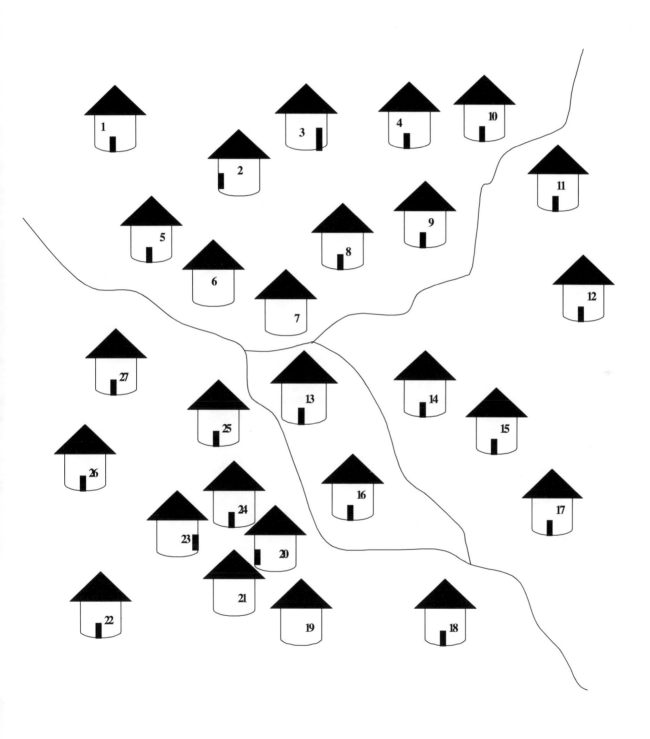

Participant's Manual, Module 3   **PM-43**

Module Three
Session 1
Overhead 3

Situation 3: Household List Not Available - Size > 30

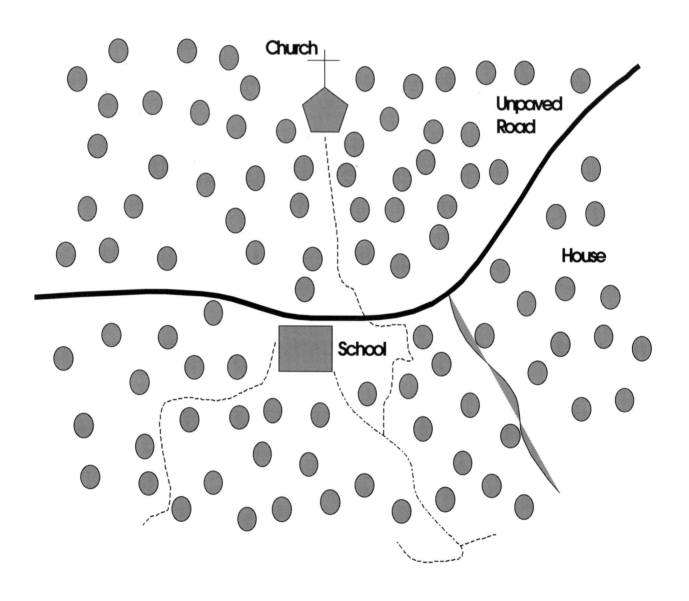

Module Three
Session 1
Overhead 4

Group of 27 Households Numbered for Random Selection of 1 Household

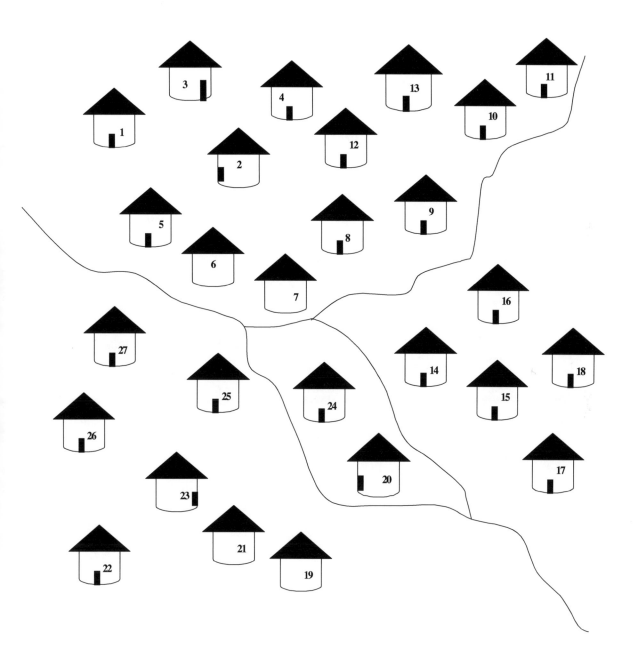

Participant's Manual, Module 3 PM-45

Module Three
Session 2
Overhead 5

Rules for Identifying Respondents

If the type of respondent you are looking for:	Then:
Is at the household* you selected	<u>Interview</u> that person <u>if</u> she consents.
Does <u>not</u> live at the household you selected	Go to the next-nearest household <u>from the front entrance</u> to the household you are at, and check at this "next-nearest" household... <u>Continue</u> this process <u>until</u> you find the respondent type you are looking for. (Hint: if 2 households are equally near, then choose the one with the closest door. Otherwise, "flip a coin.")
Lives at that household **BUT** is absent and far away (<u>more than</u> 30 minutes away)	
Lives at that household, is absent **BUT** is nearby (<u>within</u> 30 minutes)	Go <u>find</u> the respondent with the help of a guide from the community.... **IF** you <u>cannot</u> find the person in the next 30 minutes... **GO** to the next-nearest household <u>from the front entrance</u> of the household of the person you cannot find.

* <u>Household</u> = group of persons who share the same kitchen or hearth; or, a group of persons who eat from the same cooking pot.

Module Three
Session 2
Overhead 6

24 Household Composition Scenarios

- **Household #1**
  - Mother 35 years with children 6 months old and 23 months old
  - Sister of woman is 23 years old
  - Grandmother is 50 years old

- **Household #2**
  - Mother 18 years old with child 24 months, pregnant
  - Father 26 years

- **Household #3**
  - Abandoned house – owners absent

- **Household #4**
  - Girl 12 years old
  - 3-month-old baby
  - Mother of 3-month-old in market, and she is the sister of the 12-year-old
  - Mother of 6-month-old is dead, also sister of 12-year-old
  - Father in nearby field

- **Household #5**
  - Man 65 years
  - Man's wife 60 years
  - Mother of 15-month-old absent in field nearby – might be pregnant, doesn't know
  - 15-month-old baby
  - Father in city

Module Three
Session 2
Overhead 6 – Continued

- **Household #6**
  - Father 45 years old
  - One wife, 48 years old
  - Daughter, 24 years and pregnant
  - Children 2 and 3 years old

- **Household #7**
  - Mother of 9-year-old child is not home – child does not know when mother will be back
  - 9-year-old child
  - 8-month-old child of woman

- **Household #8**
  - Mother and father are not at home
  - 15-year-old girl and 16-year-old boy are present

- **Household #9**
  - 18 year old son
  - Mother of 18-year-old is 40
  - Father of 18-year-old is 70
  - 18-month-old child of mother's sister is in city

- **Household #10**
  - Woman 20 years old with child 6 months
  - Sister of 20-year-old is 25 years old and has child 3 years old
  - 3rd sister 30 years old with 12-month-old baby
  - 2 husbands, one is 25 years old, the other is 32 years – both in market playing cards

Module Three
Session 2
Overhead 6 -Continued

- ♦ **Household #11**
  - 10-year-old sister
  - 30-year-old aunt – she is pregnant
  - Woman 75 years old, mother of pregnant aunt
  - Grandfather 80 years old
  - Mother and her children in the city

- ♦ **Household #12**
  - Mother 35 years old – pregnant
  - Child of pregnant mother is 13 months old
  - Neighbor woman is 35 years old
  - Neighbor's 10-month-old baby

- ♦ **Household #13**
  - Girl 10 years old
  - 35-year-old sister of 10-year-old is at neighbor's house
  - 10-month-old baby with mother at neighbor's house

- ♦ **Household #14**
  - 8-month-old twin girls
  - Mother of twins, 27 years old
  - 40-year-old brother of mother
  - 32-year-old wife of brother (of mother)

- ♦ **Household #15**
  - New bride of 14 years with 2-month-old baby
  - Her 19-year-old husband
  - Mother-in-law 47 years
  - Husband's 26-year-old brother visiting

- ♦ **Household #16**
  - Refugee woman from neighboring country with 3-year-old
  - Her sister, who immigrated when she was 39, about 12 years ago
  - Sister's father 47 years old

Module Three

Session 2
Overhead 6 -Continued

- ◆ **Household #17**
  - Guesthouse has 42-year-old female owner who lives at the guesthouse
  - Guest: include 42-year-old businessman
  - Guest: Mother 43 years with teenage children
  - Guest: 30-year-old truck driver

- ◆ **Household #18**
  - Priest is 38 years old. He lives on the church grounds and does not maintain a separate house.
  - 42-year-old female cook also lives on the church grounds.

- ◆ **Household #19**
  - Three sisters, one with a six-week-old baby, one with an 8-month-old and one who is childless.
  - Husband of sister with 8-month-old is 24 years.

- ◆ **Household #20**
  - Mother 18 – pregnant, has 4-month-old baby
  - Father is working on the roof of the house

- ◆ **Household #21**
  - 8-year-old boy
  - His 32-year-old father is taking a shower
  - His mother, 24 years, is cooking dinner

- ◆ **Household #22**
  - Mother 18 years old with child 24 months, pregnant
  - Father 26 years

- ◆ **Household #23**
  - Abandoned house – owners absent

- ◆ **Household #24**
  - Father 45 years old
  - Wife, 35 years old and pregnant

Module Three
Session 3
Overhead 7

Process for Field Practical

1. Meet with community leader.

2. Revise and/or create community map.

3. Subdivide the community into sections of 30 or fewer households.

4. Give each section (each group of 30 or fewer households) a number.

5. Select a section using a random number.

6. Perform steps 3 through 5 again if the selected section is still too large.

7. Assign numbers to households in selected section.

8. Select a starting household using a random number table.

9. Identify the "next-nearest" household at least twice.

MODULE FOUR

What questions do I ask and how should I ask them?

Session 1: Reviewing the Survey Questionnaires
   (*no overheads needed for this section*)

Session 2: Interviewing Skills

Session 3: Field Practical for Interviewing
   (*no overheads needed for this section*)

Session 4: Planning for the Data Collection/Survey
   (*no overheads needed for this section*)
   (*handout only included in this section*)

Module Four
Session 2
Overhead 1

Why Interviewing is Important

➢ **Sound programming decisions depend on reliable data,**

and

➢ **reliable data depends on getting good information from local respondents,**

and

➢ **getting good information from respondents depends on conducting effective interviews.**

Module Four
Session 2
Overhead 2

Interview Etiquette

- **Dress appropriately.**

- **Present official document/certificate from organization or project if necessary.**

- **Be punctual (if appointments have been made).**

- **Do not enter the house unless you are invited.**

- **If you remain outside, do not ask for a chair; sit on the porch, steps, etc.**

- **Tell people how long the questionnaire will take.**

- **Do not accept lunch (unless it would be rude to refuse).**

- **Do not give gifts to interviewees.**

- **Thank interviewees at the end.**

Module Four
Session 2
Overhead 3

Effective Interviewing Techniques

1. Introduce yourself, your organization, and the purpose of the survey (show document or certificate if necessary).

2. Maintain confidentiality:
   - Do not interview the respondent in the presence of others (unless he/she indicates otherwise).
   - Explain that all answers will be kept confidential.

3. Ask questions exactly as written or with minor changes that were agreed upon during the training.

4. Wait for a response; be silent, then probe.

5. If the respondent doesn't understand or the answer is unclear, ask the question again, making as few changes in wording as possible.

6. Do not suggest—by tone of voice, facial expression, or body language—the answer you want.

7. Do not ask leading questions, questions that signal the correct answer or that suggest the answer you would like.

8. Try not to react to answers in such a way as to show that you approve or disapprove.

9. If one answer is inconsistent with another, try to clear up the confusion.

10. Try to maintain a conversational tone of voice; don't make the interview seem like an interrogation.

11. Know the local words for sensitive/delicate topics.

12. Use neutral probes (e.g., anything more?)

Module Four
Session 4
Handout for each team

Survey Checklists

1. PRE-SURVEY CHECKLIST

Before the survey begins, be sure the following tasks have been completed:

1. Review the sampling frame before designing the plan for data collection.

2. Count the questionnaires to be sure you have 19 for the respondent type and for each supervision area.

3. Number questionnaires 1 through 19 for each supervision area.

4. Review each one of the 19 questionnaires to make sure that they have the correct number of pages and they are securely stapled.

5. Review the materials checklist below. Be sure you have (or have decided you don't need) the following materials:

6. Verify questionnaires have no missing pages and are securely stapled together.

Materials Checklist

- 19 questionnaires for correct respondent + 2 extras
- Pencil
- Pencil sharpener
- Eraser
- Clipboard
- Day pack or bag to carry questionnaires and materials
- Random number tables
- Rules to select respondents in a household
- Raincoat
- Community maps or paper for making maps
- Any 'questionnaire-specific' materials: literacy tests, ORS packets, etc.)

2. CHECKLIST FOR DATA COLLECTORS

After you are in the field, make sure participants complete the survey in the following manner:

1. If a community census is available, number households and randomly select a starting household (and proceed as in step 6. below).

2. If no community census is available, update community maps, as needed, before selecting starting household(s), identifying all houses in the community. If no map is available, make one, being sure to include landmarks and showing the relative number of houses in each section of the community.

3. If the community is small, e.g., less than 30 houses, number all houses. Randomly select a starting household.

4. If the community is large, e.g., more than 30 houses, divide into sections (each section with a similar number of houses):
   - number each section;
   - randomly select one of the community sections; (If you have divided the community into 3 sections, select a random number between 1 and 3.)
   - go to the selected section to confirm the number of houses and the location of each house (and, if necessary, update the community map); if the section is large, subdivide it into subsections and randomly select one (and repeat this process until you get a subsection with 30 or fewer houses);
   - number on the map each house in the section or subsection selected;
   - randomly select one house.

5. If it is very difficult to divide the community or a section of it into sections, then:
   - ask a respondent to take you to a place where exactly 50% of the houses are in front of you, 50% of the houses are behind you, 50% are to the right and 50% are to the left;
   - number these 4 sections;
   - choose one randomly;
   - go to that section and repeat the procedure until you can see a manageable number of houses you can easily count;
   - select one of those houses randomly.

6. Go to the selected house to begin interviewing.

7. If you cannot complete an interview in the selected house, visit the closest house until the interview has been completed. Continue doing this procedure until you complete all questionnaire types as instructed.

8. After completing all questionnaire types, select another starting household (or section and then household) at random if there is more than one sampling point in the community or continue to a new community.

> *Remember: For each questionnaire, randomly select a starting household and then go to the closest house until the interview is complete.*

3. CHECKLIST FOR MANAGERS

The following is a checklist for program managers:

1. Review the data collection plan with each interviewer and supervisor.

2. Indicate the minimum number of interviews to be completed in one day.

3. During day 1 you can let data collectors work in pairs if you think this will increase their confidence.

4. Provide the technical and administrative support required by each interviewer (transport, lunch, etc.).

5. At the end of each day always review the questionnaires of each interviewer to assure that they have been correctly filled out and are complete. Check for any <u>missing</u> information or responses, and missing pages.

6. Make necessary corrections to questionnaire and inform the interviewer of problems found. If information is missing, the interviewer should revisit the house to complete the questionnaire before going to another community.

7. Confirm that all questionnaires have been filled in for each supervision area and that no pages are missing. If your LQAS sample size is 19 then you should have 19 completed questionnaires.

8. Organize the questionnaires by LQAS number (for example – from 1 to 19), according to the supervision area. For five supervision areas, for example, you would organize the questionnaires as follows:

Folder 1:   Respondent Type A, Area 1: 01 to 19
Folder 2:   Respondent Type A, Area 2: 01 to 19
Folder 3:   Respondent Type A, Area 3: 01 to 19
Folder 4:   Respondent Type A, Area 4: 01 to 19
Folder 5:   Respondent Type A, Area 5: 01 to 19

NB: Be sure to bring all the questionnaires to the tabulation workshop.

> **USE THIS MODULE TO CARRY OUT A BASELINE SURVEY FOR YOUR PROGRAM**

MODULE FIVE

What do I do with the information I have collected during baseline?

Session 1: Fieldwork Debriefing

Session 2: Tabulating Results
    (*handout*)

Session 3: Analyzing Results

Module Five
Session 1
Overhead 1

Status Report on Data Collection from the NGO or MOH Administrative Area:

NGO or MOH Administrative Area:_____

Total Supervision Areas Included in Baseline Survey = #_____

SA Number or Name	No. of Questionnaires <u>Completed</u>	No. of Questionnaires Remaining (If Any)	No. of Questionnaires Brought To The Workshop	Plan to Finish Tabulation: Dates for Data Collection, Deadline for Completion
1				
2				
3				
4				
5				
6				

Module Five
Session 2
Overhead 2

Result Tabulation Table for a Supervision Area: Baseline Survey and Regular Monitoring
Females 15 – 49 Years

Supervision Area: _____ Supervisor: _____ Date: _____

CORRECT = 1   INCORRECT = 0   SKIPPED = S   MISSING = X

#	Indicator	Correct Response Key	1	2	3	4	5	6	7	8	9	10	11	12	13	14	15	16	17	18	19	Total Correct in SA	Total Sample Size (all '0's and '1's)
Section 3: Family Planning																							
1	Age of mother at first birth	20 – 35 Years																				
2	How long should a female wait after the birth of a child to have another?	2 or more years																				
3	What can a female or male do to avoid pregnancy?	3 or more of acceptable responses (ex. 1-10)																				
Section 4: HIV/AIDS and Other Sexually Transmitted Infections																							
1	Have you ever heard of an illness called HIV/AIDS?	Yes (if No or Unknown then Quest. 3-5 automatically incorrect)																				
2	Is there anything a man can do to avoid getting HIV/AIDS?	DO NOT CODE																				
3	What can a man do to avoid getting HIV/AIDS?	2 or more acceptable responses (ex. 1-19 or 14)																				
4	Is there anything a woman can do to avoid getting HIV/AIDS?	DO NOT CODE																				
5	What can a woman do to avoid getting HIV/AIDS?	2 or more acceptable responses (ex. 1-19 or 14)																				

Module Five
Session 2
Handout for Participants

Tabulation Quality Checklist

As you tabulate your questionnaire, use the following checklist.

➤ Before You Begin:

1. Be sure the questionnaires you are about to tabulate match the type of tabulation table you have (right age, sex, etc.)

2. Confirm that questionnaires are in the correct order: 01 – 19, and confirm they have the correct number of pages.

➤ During Tabulation:

1. Work in threes.

2. The first person reads the correct answer on the tabulation sheet.

3. The second person looks at the answer on the questionnaire, determines if the answer is a "1" correct or a "0" incorrect. Mark an "S" for intentionally skipped questions that can not be judged as either correct or incorrect, and an "X" for questions that should have responses but the responses are missing. An "X" should be taken out of the denominator. An "S" should only be marked if the person should be taken out of the denominator. For example, if the question concerns a sick child but the respondent's child has not been sick, then all the questions about the sickness would be marked as "S" since they are irrelevant for this respondent. However, in most cases a skipped question is equivalent to an automatic incorrect and should be coded as "0." For example, if a respondent says he/she does not know how to prepare ORS, then all subsequent

questions related to ORS preparation would be automatically incorrect. Similarly, if a respondent does not have a vaccination card for their child, then all of the child's vaccinations would be judged as "0." On rare occasions an "S" is an automatic correct and should be coded "1."

4. The first person records the answer on the tabulation sheet.

5. The third person confirms that the second person correctly determined if the answer should be coded "1" or "0" or "S" or "X" and that the first person recorded it properly.

> **After Completing Each Column (all responses from one respondent):**

1. Check that all the marks are in the same column; there should be no marks in the column to the right of the column just completed.

2. Check that there are no blank cells in the column just completed.
- Be sure that no cells are blank. For any blank cell review the questionnaire to see if it should be coded a 0, 1, S, or X.
- Almost all responses should be a 0 or 1.
- If the cell has an "S," then check to see that it satisfies this criterion: The respondent was skipped because the question should not be asked of her/him because she/he cannot be included in the denominator. In a way, this means they are not part of the universe being assessed.

EXAMPLE 1: Some questions are asked of mothers if their child has had diarrhea in the last 2 weeks. Children who did not have diarrhea are coded "S" because the question cannot be asked of them.

EXAMPLE 2: Some questions are not asked because the questions are automatically INCORRECT or 0. If a woman is asked if she has ever heard of HIV/AIDS, and responds "No," that question is coded a 0 since it is not the desired response—it is incorrect. Any following question that asks about how HIV is transmitted or prevented would be SKIPPED since they are automatically counted as INCORRECT (coded "0") since we know the person cannot know the correct response because she does not even know that HIV exists.

- If the cell has an "X," this means the respondent should have responded to the question but for some reason no response was recorded. This could be because the interviewer forgot to do this. Sometimes an interviewer circles several responses when they should have only circled one of them. These responses are also coded as "X" since there is no clear response. Also, if you cannot decipher the response written on a questionnaire, then "X" is an appropriate code. All "Xs" are excluded from the denominator in any calculation.

3. Ask a trainer to check your tabulation sheet after you have completed the first column.

➤ After Completing a Tabulation Sheet:

1. Enter the total number correct in the appropriate column.

2. Enter the total sample size in the appropriate column.

3. Look at all questions where the sample is less than 19 and confirm the reason:

- All questions should have a "0", "1", "S", or "X." If this is not the case, find out why, so you can make an appropriate entry in the space provided.

Module Five
Session 3
Overhead 3

Summary Tabulation Table: Baseline Survey Females 15 – 49 Years

NGO name: _____ DATE: _____

#	Indicator	Total Correct in Each SA/Decision Rule						Total Correct in Program	Sample Size						Total Sample Size in Program	Average Coverage = Total Correct / Sample Size
		1	2	3	4	5	6		1	2	3	4	5	6		
Section 3: Family Planning																
1	Age of mother at first birth															
2	How long should a female wait after the birth of a child to have another?															
3	What can a female or male do to avoid pregnancy?															
Section 4: HIV/AIDS and Other Sexually Transmitted Infections																
1	Have you ever heard of an illness called HIV/AIDS?															
2	Is there anything a man can do to avoid getting HIV/AIDS?	DO NOT CODE														
3	What can a man do to avoid getting HIV/AIDS?															
4	Is there anything a woman can do to avoid getting HIV/AIDS?	DO NOT CODE														
5	What can a woman do to avoid getting HIV/AIDS?															

* To find the "Decision Rule" for each indicator, using the LQAS Table, find the "Sample Size" in the left column. Then for *baseline surveys*: look for the "Average Coverage" across the top and look down the column for the "Decision Rule." Then for *monitoring surveys*: look for the "Annual Coverage Target" across the top and look down the column for the "Decision Rule." (See Module 6.)

Module Five
Session 3
Overhead 4

LQAS Table: Decision Rules for Sample Sizes of 12-30 and Coverage Targets/Average of 10%-95%

Sample Size*	Average Coverage (Baselines) / Annual Coverage Target (Monitoring and Evaluation)																	
	10%	15%	20%	25%	30%	35%	40%	45%	50%	55%	60%	65%	70%	75%	80%	85%	90%	95%
12	N/A	N/A	1	1	2	2	3	4	5	5	6	7	7	8	8	9	10	11
13	N/A	N/A	1	1	2	3	3	4	5	6	6	7	8	8	9	10	11	11
14	N/A	N/A	1	1	2	3	4	4	5	6	7	8	8	9	10	11	11	12
15	N/A	N/A	1	2	2	3	4	5	6	6	7	8	9	10	10	11	12	13
16	N/A	N/A	1	2	2	3	4	5	6	7	8	9	9	10	11	12	13	14
17	N/A	N/A	1	2	2	3	4	5	6	7	8	9	10	11	12	13	14	15
18	N/A	N/A	1	2	2	3	5	6	7	8	9	10	11	11	12	13	14	16
19	N/A	N/A	1	2	3	4	5	6	7	8	9	10	11	12	13	14	15	16
20	N/A	N/A	1	2	3	4	5	6	7	8	9	11	12	13	14	15	16	17
21	N/A	N/A	1	2	3	4	5	6	8	9	10	11	12	13	14	16	17	18
22	N/A	N/A	1	2	3	4	5	7	8	9	10	12	13	14	15	16	18	19
23	N/A	N/A	1	2	3	4	6	7	8	10	11	12	13	14	16	17	18	20
24	N/A	N/A	1	2	3	4	6	7	9	10	11	13	14	15	16	18	19	21
25	N/A	1	2	2	4	5	6	8	9	10	12	13	14	16	17	18	20	21
26	N/A	1	2	3	4	5	6	8	9	11	12	14	15	16	18	19	21	22
27	N/A	1	2	3	4	5	7	8	10	11	13	14	15	17	18	20	21	23
28	N/A	1	2	3	4	5	7	8	10	12	13	15	16	18	19	21	22	24
29	N/A	1	2	3	4	5	7	9	10	12	13	15	17	18	20	21	23	25
30	N/A	1	2	3	4	5	7	9	11	12	14	16	17	19	20	22	24	26

N/A: *not applicable*, meaning LQAS cannot be used in this assessment because the coverage is either too low or too high to assess an SA. This table assumes the lower threshold is 30 percentage points below the upper threshold.

▨ shaded cells indicate where *alpha or beta errors are ≥ 10%*.

▥ hashed cells indicate where *alpha or beta errors are > 15%*.

Module Five
Session 3
Overhead 5

Defining Program Goals and Annual Targets

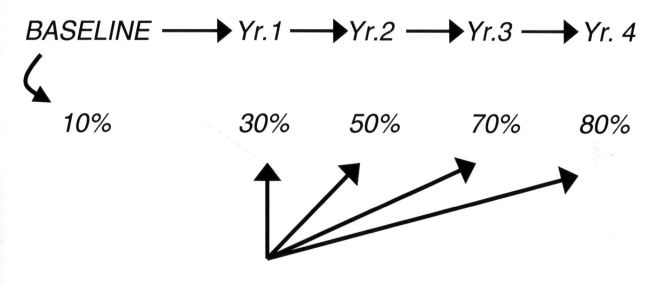

PROGRAM GOALS FROM BASELINE
UNTIL YEAR 4 OF THE PROJECT

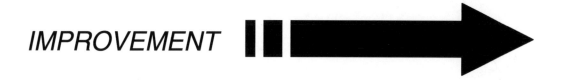

Module Five
Session 3
Overhead 6

Monitoring Targets and Average Coverage Over Time In a Catchment Area

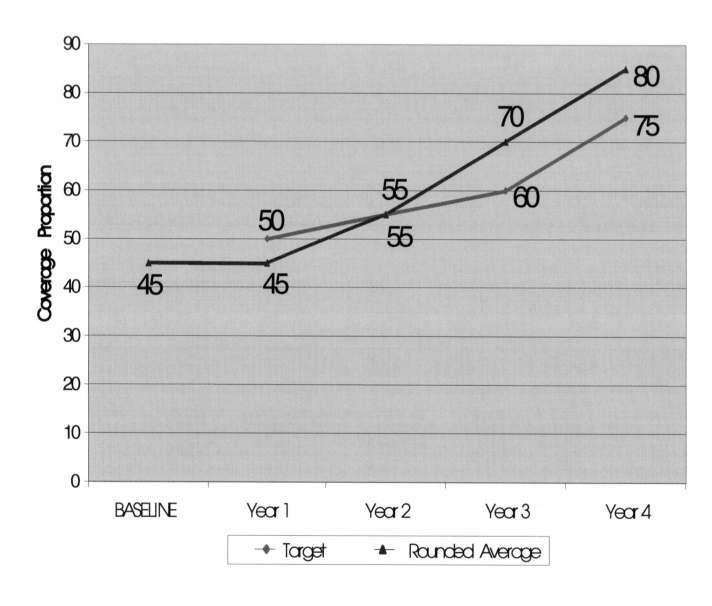

PM-68 Participant's Manual, Module 5

Module Five
Session 3
Overhead 7

How to Analyze Data and Identify Priorities Using the Summary Tables

Group Work

1. Discuss within your group the following (25 minutes):

   - **Priorities among Supervision Areas for each indicator in a group of related indicators**

   - **Priorities within one Supervision Area among a group of related indicators**

2. **Report main findings to all workshop participants (10 minutes each)**

Module Five
Session 3
Overhead 8

Baseline Survey Report Format

CONTENT	MAXIMUM PAGES (13, Excluding Appendix)
Summary	1
Program Overview (locations, objectives, main activities, beneficiaries, etc.)	1
Purpose of Baseline Survey and Methodology	1
Main Findings: Priorities by Supervision Area and for the Program as a Whole	5
Action Plans and Goals/Coverage Targets for Key Indicators	2
Conclusions and Recommendations	2
Appendix (Photocopy Summary Tabulation Tables)	1

Module Five
Session 3
Overhead 9

Methodology
(Illustrative of aspects that could be included)

➢ Training in LQAS (principles and concepts).

➢ Used a sample of 19 (randomly selected) in each Supervision Area.

➢ Number of questionnaires and questionnaire types used, which were discussed, tested and revised by NGO staff.

➢ Updated the maps in each Supervision Area with the assistance of chiefs, health workers, etc.

➢ Households were randomly chosen and, in some cases, respondents were also chosen randomly.

➢ Organization for data collection (e.g., as a group, etc.).

➢ Hand tabulation using separate tables.

Module Five
Session 3
Overhead 10

Main Findings

✓ **Priorities: Specify the program priorities by indicator, by Supervision Area and by type of respondent (e.g., men, women, and/or mothers with children of different age groups).**

For example:

The percentage of women who know danger signs during pregnancy (that indicate the need to seek care) is below average only in Supervision Areas 3 and 5. We need to focus on Areas 3 and 5 in our efforts to improve this indicator.

Among the infant and child feeding indicators, the percentage of mothers who continue to breastfeed up to and beyond 12 months of age appears to be the biggest problem (across all Supervision Areas, only 20% of mothers of children aged 12-15 months were breastfeeding at the time of the survey). This practice will receive special attention in the project's nutrition intervention.

Module Five
Session 3
Overhead 11

Action Plans and Goals/Coverage Targets for Key Indicators

➢ For each priority, list the main activities that your organization will implement to reduce the identified problems.

➢ For example, a priority activity could be to identify terms, perceived causes, preferred treatments and preferred providers for the danger signs during pregnancy that women in the community recognize. Then we can further build upon the local understanding of pregnancy danger signs to develop appropriate strategies for improving recognition and care-seeking.

➢ Report key indicators, coverage targets, and goals for your future planning.

Results of Baseline Survey, Coverage Targets, and End of Project Goals (Men 15-49 Years)

Key Indicators	Baseline Average Coverage	Projected Coverage Target Year 1	Projected Coverage Target Year 2	Projected Coverage Target Year 3	End-of-Project Goal Year 4

> **USE THIS SECTION FOR REGULAR MONITORING OF YOUR PROGRAM**

MODULE SIX

What do I do with the information I have collected during monitoring?

Session 1: Fieldwork Debriefing

Session 2: Tabulating Results
(*handout*)

Session 3: Analyzing Results

Module Six
Session 1
Overhead 1

Status Report on Data Collection from the NGO or MOH Administrative Area:

NGO or MOH Administrative Area: _____

Total Supervision Areas Included in Monitoring Survey = #_____

SA Number or Name	No. of Questionnaires <u>Completed</u>	No. of Questionnaires Remaining (If Any)	No. of Questionnaires Brought To The Workshop	Plan to Finish Tabulation: Dates for Data Collection, Deadline for Completion
1				
2				
3				
4				
5				
6				

Module Six
Session 2
Overhead 2

Result Tabulation Table for a Supervision Area: Baseline Survey and Regular Monitoring
Females 15 – 49 Years

Supervision Area: _____ Supervisor: _____ Date: _____

CORRECT = 1 INCORRECT = 0 SKIPPED = S MISSING = X

#	Indicator	Correct Response Key	1	2	3	4	5	6	7	8	9	10	11	12	13	14	15	16	17	18	19	Total Correct in SA	Total Sample Size (all '0's and '1's)
Section 3: Family Planning																							
1	Age of mother at first birth	20 – 35 Years																					
2	How long should a female wait after the birth of a child to have another?	2 or more years																					
3	What can a female or male do to avoid pregnancy?	3 or more of acceptable responses (ex. 1-10)																					
Section 4: HIV/AIDS and Other Sexually Transmitted Infections																							
1	Have you ever heard of an illness called HIV/AIDS?	Yes (if No or Unknown then Quest. 3-5 automatically incorrect)																					
2	Is there anything a man can do to avoid getting HIV/AIDS?	DO NOT CODE																					
3	What can a man do to avoid getting HIV/AIDS?	2 or more acceptable responses (ex. 1-19 or 14)																					
4	Is there anything a woman can do to avoid getting HIV/AIDS?	DO NOT CODE																					
5	What can a woman do to avoid getting HIV/AIDS?	2 or more acceptable responses (ex. 1-19 or 14)																					

Module Six
Session 2
Handout for Participants

Tabulation Quality Checklist

As you tabulate your questionnaire, use the following checklist.

➢ Before You Begin:

1. Be sure the questionnaires you are about to tabulate match the type of tabulation table you have (right age, sex, etc.)

2. Confirm that questionnaires are in the correct order: 01-19, and that they have the correct number of pages.

➢ During Tabulation:

1. Work in threes.

2. The first person reads the correct answer on the tabulation sheet.

3. The second person looks at the answer on the questionnaire, determines if the answer is a "1" correct or a "0" incorrect. Mark an "S" for intentionally skipped questions that can <u>not</u> be judged as either correct or incorrect, and an "X" for questions that should have responses but the responses are missing. An "X" should be taken out of the denominator. An "S" should only be marked if the person should be taken out of the denominator. For example, if the question concerns a sick child but the respondent's child has not been sick, then all the questions about the sickness would be marked as "S" since they are irrelevant for this respondent. However, in most cases a skipped question is equivalent to an automatic incorrect and should be coded as "0." For example, if a respondent says they do not know how to prepare ORS, then all subsequent

questions related to ORS preparation would be automatically incorrect. Similarly, if a respondent does not have a vaccination card for their child, then all of the child's vaccinations would be judged as "0." On rare occasions it is an automatic correct and should be coded "1."

4. The first person records the answer on the tabulation sheet.

5. The third person confirms that the second person correctly determined if the answer should be coded "1" or "0" or "S" or "X" and that the first person recorded it properly.

➤ After Completing Each Column (all responses from one respondent):

1. Check that all the marks are in the same column; there should be no marks in the column to the right of the column just completed.

2. Check that there are no blank cells in the column just completed.
   - Be sure that no cells are blank. For any blank cell, review the questionnaire to see if it should be coded a 0, 1, S, or X.
   - Almost all responses should be a 0 or 1.
   - If the cell has an "S," then check to see that it satisfies this criterion: The respondent was skipped because the question should not be asked of her/him because she/he cannot be included in the denominator. In a way, this means they are not part of the universe being assessed.

   EXAMPLE 1: Some questions are asked of mothers if their child has had diarrhea in the last 2 weeks. Children who did not have diarrhea are coded "S" because the question cannot be asked of them.

EXAMPLE 2: Some questions are not asked because the questions are automatically INCORRECT or 0. If a women is asked if she has ever heard of HIV/AIDS, and responds "No," that question is coded a 0 since it is not the desired response – it is incorrect. Any following question that asks questions about how HIV is transmitted or prevented would be SKIPPED since they are automatically counted as INCORRECT (coded "0") since we know the person cannot know the correct response because she does not even know that HIV exists.

- If the cell has an "X," this means the respondent should have responded to the question but for some reason no response was recorded. This could be because the interviewer forgot to do this. Sometimes an interviewer circles several responses when they should have only circled one of them. These responses are also coded as "X" since there is no clear response. Also, if you cannot decipher the response written on a questionnaire, then "X" is an appropriate code. All "Xs" are excluded from the denominator in any calculation.

3. Ask a trainer to check your tabulation sheet after you have completed the first column.

➢ After Completing a Tabulation Sheet:

1. Enter the total number correct in the appropriate column.

2. Enter the total sample size in the appropriate column.

3. Look at all questions where the sample is less than 19 and confirm the reason:

- All questions should have a "0", "1", "S", or "X." If this is not the case, find out why, so you can make an appropriate entry in the space provided.

Module Six
Session 3
Overhead 3

Summary Tabulation Table: Regular Monitoring Females 15 – 49 Years

NGO name: _____   DATE: _____

#	Indicator	Total Correct in Each SA/Decision Rule						Total Correct in Program	Sample Size						Total Sample Size in Program	Average Coverage = Total Correct / Sample Size	Coverage Target
		1	2	3	4	5	6		1	2	3	4	5	6			

CIRCLE IF BELOW AVERAGE COVERAGE DECISION RULE — **MARK WITH A STAR (*) IF BELOW COVERAGE TARGET DECISION RULE**

Section 3: Family Planning

#	Indicator	1	2	3	4	5	6	Total Correct in Program	1	2	3	4	5	6	Total Sample Size in Program	Average Coverage	Coverage Target
1	Age of mother at first birth																
2	How long should a female wait after the birth of a child to have another?																
3	What can a female or male do to avoid pregnancy?																

Section 4: HIV/AIDS and Other Sexually Transmitted Infections

#	Indicator	1	2	3	4	5	6	Total Correct in Program	1	2	3	4	5	6	Total Sample Size in Program	Average Coverage	Coverage Target
1	Have you ever heard of an illness called HIV/AIDS?																
2	Is there anything a man can do to avoid getting HIV/AIDS?	DO NOT CODE															
3	What can a man do to avoid getting HIV/AIDS?																
4	Is there anything a woman can do to avoid getting HIV/AIDS?	DO NOT CODE															
5	What can a woman do to avoid getting HIV/AIDS?																

Module Six
Session 3
Overhead 4

LQAS Table: Decision Rules for Sample Sizes of 12-30 and Coverage Targets/Average of 10%-95%

Sample Size*	Average Coverage (Baselines) / Annual Coverage Target (Monitoring and Evaluation)																	
	10%	15%	20%	25%	30%	35%	40%	45%	50%	55%	60%	65%	70%	75%	80%	85%	90%	95%
12	N/A	N/A	1	1	2	2	3	4	5	5	6	7	7	8	8	9	10	11
13	N/A	N/A	1	1	2	3	3	4	5	6	6	7	8	8	9	10	11	11
14	N/A	N/A	1	1	2	3	4	4	5	6	7	8	8	9	10	11	11	12
15	N/A	N/A	1	2	2	3	4	5	6	6	7	8	9	10	10	11	12	13
16	N/A	N/A	1	2	2	3	4	5	6	7	8	9	9	10	11	12	13	14
17	N/A	N/A	1	2	2	3	4	5	6	7	8	9	10	11	11	12	13	15
18	N/A	N/A	1	2	2	3	5	6	7	8	8	10	11	11	12	13	14	16
19	N/A	N/A	1	2	3	4	5	6	7	8	9	10	11	12	13	14	15	16
20	N/A	N/A	1	2	3	4	5	6	7	8	9	11	12	13	14	15	16	17
21	N/A	N/A	1	2	3	4	5	6	8	9	10	11	12	13	14	16	17	18
22	N/A	N/A	1	2	3	4	5	7	8	9	10	12	13	14	15	16	18	19
23	N/A	N/A	1	2	3	4	6	7	8	10	11	12	13	14	16	17	18	20
24	N/A	N/A	1	2	3	4	6	7	9	10	11	13	14	15	16	18	19	21
25	N/A	1	2	2	4	5	6	8	9	10	12	13	14	16	17	18	20	21
26	N/A	1	2	3	4	5	6	8	9	11	12	14	15	16	18	19	21	22
27	N/A	1	2	3	4	5	7	8	10	11	13	14	15	17	18	20	21	23
28	N/A	1	2	3	4	5	7	8	10	12	13	15	16	18	19	21	22	24
29	N/A	1	2	3	4	5	7	9	10	12	13	15	17	18	20	21	23	25
30	N/A	1	2	3	4	5	7	9	11	12	14	16	17	19	20	22	24	26

N/A: *not applicable*, meaning LQAS cannot be used in this assessment because the coverage is either too low or too high to assess an SA. This table assumes the lower threshold is 30 percentage points below the upper threshold.

▨ : shaded cells indicate where *alpha* or *beta* errors are ≥ 10%.
▨ : hashed cells indicate where *alpha* or *beta* errors are > 15%.

Module Six
Session 3
Overhead 5

Defining Program Goals and Annual Targets

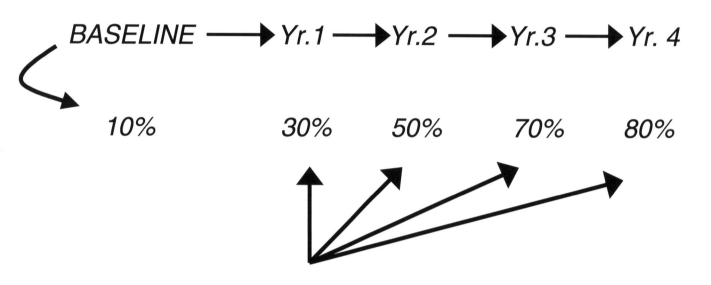

PROGRAM GOALS FROM BASELINE UNTIL YEAR 4 OF THE PROJECT

IMPROVEMENT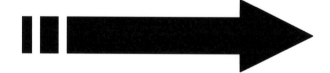

Module Six
Session 3
Overhead 6

How to Identify Priority Supervision Areas Using the Summary Tables During Regular Monitoring

SA Classification Results		Priority Status
Below the Coverage Target	Below Average	Highest
Below the Coverage Target	Not Below Average	Second Highest
Not Below the Coverage Target	Below Average	Second Highest
Not Below the Coverage Target	Not Below Average	Not a Priority

Participant's Manual, Module 6   **PM-83**

Module Six
Session 3
Overhead 7

Using LQAS to Assess One Indicator Over the Life of a Project

	BASE-LINE	Year 1	Year 2	Year 3	Year 4
Target		50	55	60	75
Decision Rule		7	8	9	12
Rounded Average	45	45	55	70	80
Decision Rule	6	6	8	11	13
SA 1	12	13	14	12	(12)
SA 2	7	6*	(7*)	14	(12)
SA 3	6	9	12	11	17
SA 4	10	11	11	(10)	13
SA 5	(5)	(5*)	10	14	16
SA 6	6	(5*)	11	15	18
Average	40.4%	43.0%	50.9%	66.7%	77.2%

Which SAs are below average?
... and which have reached the coverage target?

Module Six
Session 3
Overhead 8

Monitoring Targets and Average Coverage Over Time In a Catchment Area

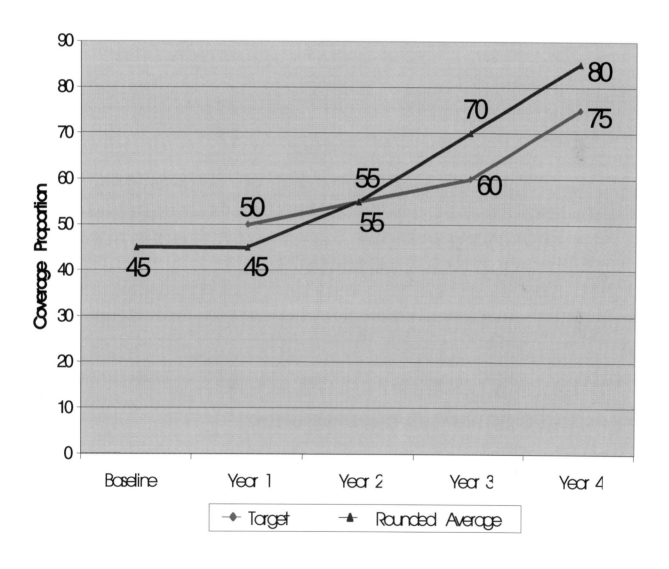

Participant's Manual, Module 6   **PM-85**

Module Six
Session 3
Overhead 9

How to Analyze Data and Identify Priorities Using the Summary Tables

Group Work

1. Discuss within your group the following (25 minutes):

   - Priorities <u>among</u> Supervision Areas for each indicator in a group of related indicators

   - Priorities <u>within one</u> Supervision Area among a group of related indicators

2. Report main findings to all workshop participants (10 minutes each)

Module Six
Session 3
Overhead 10

Monitoring Survey Report Format

CONTENT	MAXIMUM PAGES (13, Excluding Appendix)
Summary	1
Program Overview (locations, objectives, main activities, beneficiaries, etc.)	1
Purpose of Monitoring Survey and Methodology	1
Main Findings: Accomplishments, Priorities by Supervision Area and for the Program as a Whole	5
Action Plans and Goals/Coverage Targets for Key Indicators	2
Conclusions and Recommendations	2
Appendix (Photocopy Summary Tabulation Tables)	1

Module Six
Session 3
Overhead 11

Methodology
(Illustrative of aspects that could be included)

➤ Training in LQAS (principles and concepts).

➤ Used a sample of 19 (randomly selected) in each Supervision Area.

➤ Number of questionnaires and questionnaire types used, which were discussed, tested and revised by NGO staff.

➤ Updated the maps in each Supervision Area with the assistance of chiefs, health workers, etc.

➤ Households were randomly chosen and, in some cases, respondents were also chosen randomly.

➤ Organization for data collection (e.g., as a group, etc.).

➤ Hand tabulation using separate tables.

Module Six
Session 3
Overhead 12

Main Findings

✓ **Priorities: Specify the program priorities by indicator, by Supervision Area and by type of respondent (e.g., men, women, and/or mothers with children of different age groups).**

For example:

The percentage of women who know danger signs during pregnancy (that indicate the need to seek care) is below average only in Supervision Areas 3 and 5. We need to focus on Areas 3 and 5 in our efforts to improve this indicator.

Among the infant and child feeding indicators, the percentage of mothers who continue to breastfeed up to and beyond 12 months of age appears to be the biggest problem (across all Supervision Areas, only 20% of mothers of children aged 12-15 months were breastfeeding at the time of the survey). This practice will receive special attention in the project's nutrition intervention.

Module Six
Session 3
Overhead 13

Action Plans and Goals/Coverage Targets for Key Indicators

➢ For each priority, list the main activities that your organization will implement to reduce the identified problems.

➢ For example, a priority activity could be to identify terms, perceived causes, preferred treatments and preferred providers for the danger signs during pregnancy that women in the community recognize. Then we can further build upon the local understanding of pregnancy danger signs to develop appropriate strategies for improving recognition and care seeking .

➢ Report key indicators, coverage targets, and goals for your future planning. Revise coverage targets as needed.

Results of Monitoring Survey, Coverage Targets, and End of Project Goals (Men 15-49 Years)

Key Indicators	Baseline Average Coverage	Year 1 Coverage		Projected Coverage Target Year 2	Projected Coverage Target Year 3	End of Project Goal Year 4
		Observed	Target			

Bring This Table With You to Use in the Field or for Easy Reference.

LQAS Table: Decision Rules for Sample Sizes of 12-30 and Coverage Targets/Average of 10%-95%

Sample Size*	Average Coverage (Baselines) / Annual Coverage Target (Monitoring and Evaluation)																	
	10%	15%	20%	25%	30%	35%	40%	45%	50%	55%	60%	65%	70%	75%	80%	85%	90%	95%
12	N/A	N/A	1	1	2	2	3	4	5	5	6	7	7	8	8	9	10	11
13	N/A	N/A	1	1	2	3	3	4	5	6	6	7	8	8	9	10	11	11
14	N/A	N/A	1	1	2	3	4	4	5	6	7	8	8	9	10	11	11	12
15	N/A	N/A	1	2	2	3	4	5	6	6	7	8	9	10	10	11	12	13
16	N/A	N/A	1	2	2	3	4	5	6	7	8	9	9	10	10	12	13	14
17	N/A	N/A	1	2	2	3	4	5	6	7	8	9	10	11	11	13	14	15
18	N/A	N/A	1	2	2	3	5	6	7	8	9	10	11	11	12	13	14	16
19	N/A	N/A	1	2	3	4	5	6	7	8	9	10	11	12	13	14	15	16
20	N/A	N/A	1	2	3	4	5	6	7	8	9	11	12	13	14	15	16	17
21	N/A	N/A	1	2	3	4	5	6	8	9	10	11	12	13	14	16	17	18
22	N/A	N/A	1	2	3	4	5	7	8	9	10	12	13	14	15	16	18	19
23	N/A	N/A	1	2	3	4	6	7	8	10	11	12	13	14	16	17	18	20
24	N/A	N/A	1	2	3	4	6	7	9	10	11	13	14	15	16	18	19	21
25	N/A	1	2	2	4	5	6	8	9	10	12	13	14	16	17	18	20	21
26	N/A	1	2	3	4	5	6	8	9	11	12	14	15	16	18	19	21	22
27	N/A	1	2	3	4	5	7	8	10	11	13	14	15	17	18	20	21	23
28	N/A	1	2	3	4	5	7	8	10	12	13	15	16	18	19	21	22	24
29	N/A	1	2	3	4	5	7	9	10	12	13	15	17	18	20	21	23	25
30	N/A	1	2	3	4	5	7	9	11	12	14	16	17	19	20	22	24	26

N/A: *not applicable*, meaning LQAS can not be used in this assessment because the coverage is either too low or too high to assess an SA. This table assumes the lower threshold is 30 percentage points below the upper threshold.

▦ : shaded cells indicate where *alpha* or *beta* errors are ≥ 10%.
▨ : hashed cells indicate where *alpha* or *beta* errors are > 15%.